MIGR

CW00663928

And its

HOMOEOPATHIC TREATMENT

By
S. J. L. Mount, M.B.,
M.R.C.P. F. F. Hom

B. Jain Publishers P. Ltd.

Reprint edition : 2004

Price. Rs. 19.00

Published by

Kuldeep Jain

for

B. Jain Publishers (P) Ltd.

1921, Chuna Mandi, St. 10th Paharganj,
New Delhi-110 055
Phones: 2358 0800, 2358 1100, 2358 1300, 2358 3100
Fax: 011-2358 0471   *Email:* bjain@vsnl.com
Website: **www.bjainbooks.com**

PRINTED IN INDIA
by
Unisons Techno Financial Consultants (P) Ltd.
522, FIE, Patpar Ganj, Delhi-110 092

ISBN: 81-7021-552-8
BOOK CODE: B-3753

Publisher's Note

It is said that around one person in ten has migraine headaches round the world, with women being affected about three times as often as men. The pain and other symptoms may be so severe that sufferers are incapacited for several hours a day as long as the attack lasts. Although it is recognized as one of the most intractable diseases, drug treatment has a lot to offer both in preventing attacks and in shortening them when they occur. This is an exhaustive thesis on the genesis, nature and control of Migraine with particular reference to the bowel nosodes as expounded by Dr. John paterson and the homoeopathic remedies which have proved their efficacy in the treatment of migraine. We do hope that this treatise will be found useful alike by the profession and the lay public.

* * *

MIGRAINE

Historical Introduction

Migraine affects a substantial minority of the population, occurs in all civilisations, and has been recognised since the dawn of recorded history. If it was a scourge or an encouragement to Caesar, Paul Kant and Freund, it is also a daily fact of life to anonymous millions who suffer in secrecy and silence. Its forms and symptoms, as Burton remarked of melancholy, are "irregular, obscure, various, so infinite, Proteus himself is not so diverse". Its nature and causes puzzled Hippocrates and have been the subject of argument for two thousand years.

The major clinical characterstics of migraine-its periodicity, its relation to diet and circumstances, its physical and emotional symptoms- had all been clearly recognised by the second century of our era. Thus Aretaeus describes it, under the name of heterocrania:

"And in certain cases the whole head is pained and the pain is sometimes on the right and sometimes on the left side, or the forehead, or the fontanelle; and such attacks shift their place during the same day .... This is called heterocrania, an illness by no means mild. It occasions unseemly and dreadful symptoms .... nausea, vomiting of bilious matters; collapse of the patient. . there is much torpor, heaviness of the head, anxiety and life becomes a burden. For they flee the light; the darkness soothes their disease; nor can they bear readily to look upon or hear anything pleasant .... The patients are weary of life and wish to die".

While his contemporary Pelops described and named the sensory symptoms which might precede an epilepsy (the aura), Aretaeus observed the analogous symptoms which inaugurated certain migraines:

" ...... flashes of purple or black colours before the sight, or all mixed together so as to exhibit the appearance of a rainbow expended in the heavens."

1400 years elapsed between the observations of Aretaeus and the treatises of Alexander Trallianus. Throughout this period repeated observations confirmed and elaborated the terse description of Aretaeus, while reiterating unquestioned, the theories of antiquity concerning its nature. The terms heterocrania, holocrania and hemicrania, struggled with each other for many centuries; hemicrania ousted its rivals and has finally evolved, through an immense number of transliterations, to the migraine or megrin we speak of today. The terms 'sick headache', 'bilious headache' (cephalia biliosa) and 'blind headache' have been in popular use for many centuries.

Two categories of theory have dominated medical thinking on the nature of migraine since the time of Hippocrates; both were still a matter of serious dispute at the end of the 18th century and both, variously transformed, command wide popular assent today: the humoral theroy and the sympathetic theory.

An excess of yellow or black bile, it was supposed, could occasion not only a liverish feeling, black humour, or a jaundiced view of life, but the bilious vomiting and gastric upset of a sick headache. The essence of this theory and of the form of treatment which it implies, is precisely expressed by Alexander Trallianus:

"If therefore headache frequently arises on account of a superfluity of bilious humour, the cure of it must be effected by means of remedies which purge and draw away the bilious humour."

Purging and drawing away the bilious humour—in this lies the historical justification of innumerable derivative theories and treatments, many of them practised at the present day. The stomach and bowel may become laden with bilious humours; hence the time-honoured use of emetics, laxatives, cathartics, purgatives, etc. Fatty foods draw bilious humours to the stomach, therefore, the diet of the migrainer must be sparse and ascetic. Thus Fothergilla, a life-long sufferer from migraine, considered the following especially dangerous:

"Melted butter, fat meats, spices, meat-pies hot buttered toast and malt liquors when strong and happy ...."

Similarly, it has always been considered and is still so held, that constipation (i.e. retention of bilious humours in the bowel) may provoke or prelude an attack of migraine. Similarly bilious humours might be reduced at source (a variety of liver pills is still recommended for migraine), or diminished if their concentration in the blood become too high (blood-letting was particularly recommended in the 16th and 17th centuries as cure for migraine).

Contemporary in origin with the humoral theories, and evolving concurrently with them, have been a variety of "sympathetic" theories. These hold that migraine has a peripheral origin in one or more of the viscera (the stomach, the bowel, the uterus, etc.) from which it is propagated about the body by a special form of internal, visceral communication; this occult form of communication, hidden from and below the transactions of consciousness, was termed "sympathy" by the Greeks, and "consensus" by the Romans, and was conceived to be of particular importance in connecting the head and the viscera *("mirum inter caput et viscera commercium").*

The classical notions of sympathy were revived and given a more exact form by Thomas Willis. Willis had come to reject the Hippocratic notions of hysteria as arising from the physical trajectory of the womb about the body and instead came to visualize the uterus as radiating the phenomena of hysteria through an infinitude of minute pathways about the body. He extended this concept to the transmission of a migraine throughout the body and of many other paroxysmal disorders.

Willis set out three centuries ago to review the entire domain of nervous disorders (Dr. Annima Brutorum) and in the course of this work included a section (De Cephalalgia) which must be considered as the first modern treatise on migraine, and the first decisive advance since the time of Aretaeus. He organised a vast mass of medieval observations and speculations on the subject of migraine, epilepsy and the other paroxysmal reactions, and added to these clinical observations which are extraordinary in the accuracy and sobriety.

Willis, discussing migraine, shows himself fully aware of the many predisposing, exciting and accessory causes of such attacks. "........ An evil or weak constitution of the parts ...... sometimes the hereditary .... an irritation in some distant member of viscera ...... changes of season, atmospheric states, the great aspects of the sun and moon, violent passions, and errors in diet." He was well aware, also, that migraine though frequently intolerable, is benign.

A classical concept revived by Willis was that of "idiopathy" a tendency to periodic and sudden explosions in the nervous system.

Thus the migraine nervous system, or the epileptic nervous system, could be detonated at any time, by a variety of influences — physical or emotional — and the remotest effects of the explosion were conveyed throughout the body by sympathy, by presumed sympathetic nerves whose existence Willis himself could only infer. This concept is very close to the syndrome picture that Paterson correlated with Proteus.

Sympathetic theories were particularly favoured and elaborated in the 18th century. Tissot, observing that stomach disorders might precede and apparently inaugurate a migraine headache, and that vomiting could rapidly bring the entire attack to a close suggests:

"it is then most probable that a focus of irritation is formed little by little in the stomach, and that when it has reached certain point, the irritation is sufficient to give rise to acute pains in all the ramifications of the supraorbital nerve........."

"Contemporary with Tissot, and also lending the weight of his authority to such sympathetic theories was Robert Whytt; observing .... the vomiting that generally accompanies inflammation of the womb; the nausea, the disordered appetite, that follows conception........ the headache, the head and pains in the back, the intestinal colic suffered when the time of the menstrual flow approaches........ etc".

Whytt pictures the human body as riddled, from one extremity to another by obscure but strangely direct paths of sympathy; paths which could transmit the phenomena of a migraine, or a hysteria, from their visceral origins.

It is important to note that the finest clinical observers of the 18th century — Tissot, Whytt, Sydenham, etc. — made no arbitrary distinctions between physical and emotional symptoms: all had to be considered together as integral parts of "nervous disorders". Thus Robert Whytt brings together, as intimate and inter-related symptoms:

> "........ An extraordinary sensation of cold and heat, of pains in several parts of the body; syncopes and vaporous convulsions; catalepsy and tetanus; gas in the stomach and intestine ...... vomiting of black matter; a sudden and abundant flow of clear pale urine .... palpitations of the heart; variations in the pulse; periodic headaches; vertigo and nervous spells.....depression, despair ..... madness and nightmares.

This central belief, this concept of the inseparable unity of psycho-physiological reactions, was fractured at the start of the 19th century The "nervous disorders" of Willis and Whytt were rigidly divided into "organic" versus "functional". Living and Jackson, however, portrayed migraine as an indivisible psycho-physiological entity without internal divisions, but their views were conceptional and against the bias of their century.

Homoeopathy can valuably contribute to this approach whereby the whole body is seen as a single functioning unit, where a man's psychological aspect is part of his physiological state and body and mind are not divorced.

At the end of the 18th century, theories and writings on migraine dwelt on the physical aspects of migraine attacks, while neglecting their emotional components, antecedents, and uses. The theories of the 19th century, likewise, lacked the generality of the earlier doctrines and were usually concerned with very specific mechanical aetiologies of one type or another. Vascular theories were very popular, whether these envisaged general plethora, cerebral congestion, or specific dilatations and constrictions of the cranial vessels. Local factors were given great weight, swelling of the pituitary gland, inflammation in the eyes, etc.

Edward Living's treatise on Megrim, Sick Headache and Allied Disorders, published in 1873, is a remarkably penetrating work and contains much valuable comment on migraine. An essential part of Living's vision (and in this he was more related to Willis and Whytt than to his contemporaries) was the realisation that the varieties of migraine were endless in number and that they coalesced with many other paroxysmal reactions. His own theory of "nerve-storms" of great generality and power, explained, as no other theory could, the sudden or gradual metamorphosis so characteristic of migraine, faints, vagal attacks, vertigo, sleep disorders, etc., as related to each other and to epilepsy-all such nerve-storms being mutually if mysteriously transformable amongst themselves.

The present century has been characterised both by advances and retrogressions in its approach to migraine. The advances reflect sophistications of technique and the retrogressions represent the splitting and fracturing of the subject which appears inseparable from the specialization of knowledge. By a historical irony, a real gain of knowledge and technical skill has been coupled with a real loss in general understanding.

A migraine is a physical event which may also be from

the start, or later become, an emotional or symbolic event. A migraine expresses both physiological and emotional needs; it is the prototype of psycho-physiological reaction. To understand it demands a convergence of thinking which must be based, simultaneously, both on neurology and on psychiatry finally; migraine cannot be conceived as an exclusively human reaction, but must be considered as a form of biological reaction specifically tailored to human needs and human nervous systems. For this purpose migraine must be seen as an attempt on the part of the body to heal itself, to achieve balance and find harmony. The "disease" precedes the migrainous attack, while the attack itself is the "healing" reaction.

The Nature of Migraine

The cardinal symptoms of common migraine are headache and nausea. Complementing these may be a remarkable variety of other major symptoms, in addition to major disorders and physiological changes of which the patient may not be aware. Presiding over the entire attack there will be, in du Bois Reymonds' words "a general feeling of disorder", which may be experienced in either physical or emotional terms, and tax or elude the patient's powers of description. Great variability of symptoms is characteristic, not only of attacks in different patients, but between successive attacks in the same patient.

Headache —   The character of the pains varied very
              much; most frequently they were of a
              hammering, throbbing or pushing nature
              ... (in other cases) pressing and dull.......
              boring with sense of bursting ...... pricking,
              rending .... stretching .... piercing ......
              and radiating .... in a few cases it is felt

as if a wedge was pressed into the head,
or like an ulcer, or as if the brain was torn,
or pressed outwards.

Peters, 1853

Migraine headache is traditionally described as a violent throbbing pain in one temple and not infrequently takes this form. It is impossible, however, to specify a constant site, quality, or intensity, for in the course of practice one will encounter all conceivable varieties of head pain in the context of migraine. Wolff has stated (1963):

The sites of the migraine headache are notably temporal, supraorbital, frontal, retrobulbar, parietal, postauricular, and occipital .... They may occur as well in the malar region, in the upper and the lower teeth wall of the orbit, in the neck and in the region of the common carotid arteries, and down as far as the tip of the shoulder.

One may say, however that migraine headache is unilateral in onset more frequently than not, although it tends to become diffused in distribution later in the attack. One side is generally attacked by preference and in a few patients, there may be in invariable left - or right - sided involvement throughout life. More commonly there is only a relative preference, often associated with the severity of pain: severe frequent hemicrania on one side with mild occasional hemicrania on the opposite side in successive attacks, or even in the same attack.

The quality of migraine headache is similarly variable. Throbbing occurs in less than half of all cases, and in these may characterize the headache only at its inception, soon giving way to a steady aching. Continued throbbing throughout the attack is uncommon, and occurs chiefly in those who drive themselves to continued physical activity despite a migraine. Throbbing when it occurs is synchronized with arterial pulsation, and may be accompanied by visible pulsation of extracranial arteries. One may say, however, that almost all vascular headaches are aggravated by active or passive head-movement, or by the transmitted impulse of coughing, sneezing or vomiting. The pain is therefore, minimized by rest, or by splitting of the head in one position. It may also be mollified by counter pressure; many migraine sufferers will press the affected temple into their pillows, or hold the affected side with their hand.

The duration of migraine headache is very variable. In extremely acute attacks ("migrainous neuralgia") the pain may last only a matter of minutes. In a common migraine the duration is rarely less than three hours, is commonly of 8-24 hours' duration and on occasion may last several days, or in excess of a week. Tissue changes may become manifest in very extended attacks. The superficial temporal artery (or arteries) may become indurated. The surrounding skin may also become tender, and remain in this state for more than a day following the subsidence of the headache. Very rarely a spontaneous hygroma or haematoma may form about the affected vessel.

The intensity of migrainous headache is extremely variable. It may be of incapacitating violence, or so faint that its presence is only detected by the transient pain consequent upon jolting of the head on coughing. Nor need the intensity remain constant throughout the attack; a slow waxing and waning with a period of a few minutes is commonly described, and much longer remissions and exacerbations may also occur, particularly in protracted menstrual migraines.

Migrainous headache is frequently complicated by the simultaneous or antecedent occurrence of other types of head-pain. Characteristic "tension-headache", localized specially in the cervical and posterior occipital regions, may inaugurate a migraine headache, or accompany it, particularly, if the attack is marked by irritability, anxiety, or continued activity throughout its duration. Such tension-headache must not be construed as an integral portion of the migraine, but as a secondary reaction to it.

Conversely a cervical osteopathic lesion can cause a migraine and the physician should be well aware of this possibility and arrange to have a migraine patient examined by a suitably qualified colleague for such a lesion.

Homoeopathic remedies associated with the headache as such, include Belladonna, Bryonia, Glonoine. Nat.Mur., Nux Vomica, Sanguinaria, Silicea, Spigelia, Iris, Pulsatilla, Gelsemium, Lachesis, Sepia.

Nausea and associated symptoms.

Eructations occur, either inodorous and without taste, or of an insupportable mawkishness; abundant mucosities and salivary fluid flow into the mouth, intermixed at times with those of a bitter, bilious taste; there is extreme disgust for food; general malaise ..... paroxysmal distensions of the stomach with gas, followed by belchings, with transient relief; or vomiting may occur...... *(Peters, 1853)*

Nausea is invariable in the course of a common migraine, whether it is trifling and intermittent, continuous and overwhelming. The term "nausea" is used and has always been used, in both literal and figurative senses, as denoting not only a specific (if unlocalizable) sensation, but a state of mind and pattern of behaviour—a turning away from food, from every thing and a turning-inwards. Even if there is no overt nausea, a vast majority of migraine patients will be averse to eating during the attack, knowing that the act of eating, the sight, the smell, of even the very thought of food may bring on overwhelming nausea. One might almost speak of latent nausea in this connection.

A variety of other symptoms, local and systemic, are likely to be associated wih nausea. Increased salivation and reflux of bitter stomach contents (waterbrash), with the necessity of swallowing or spitting may not only accompany the sensation of nausea, but precede it by several minutes.

Not uncommonly patients are alerted to the imminence of severe sick headache by finding their mouths filled with saliva or waterbrash and may be enabled, by this timely signal, to take appropriate medication and ward off further oncoming symptoms.

Established nausea provokes various forms of visceral ejaculation: hiccup, belching, retching and vomiting. If the patient is fortunate, vomiting may terminate not only his nausea but the entire migraine attack: more commonly he will fail to secure relief from vomiting, and suffer instead an excruciating aggravation of concurrent vascular headache. When florid, nausea is far less tolerable than headache or other forms of pain, and in many patients, especially youthful ones, nausea and vomiting dominate the clinical picture and constitute the crowning misery of a common migraine.

Repeated vomiting first empties the existing stomach contents; is followed by vomiting of regurgitated bile, and finally by repeated "dry"heaving or retching. It is the chief cause (in company with profuse sweating and diarrhoea) of the severe fluid and electrolyte depletion which can prostrate patients suffering protracted attacks.

Nausea as a homoeopathic symptom in migraine is associated with such remedies as Nux vomica, Sepia, Arg.nit., Bryonia, Ipecacuaunha, Iris, Sanguinaria.

The picturesque terms "red migraine" and "white migraine" were introduced by Du-Bois Reymond, and retain a certain descriptive value. In a red migraine the face is dusky and flushed; in the words of an old account:

> congested, with rushing and roaring in the head, bloating, glowing and shining of the face, with protrusion of the eyes .....great heat of the head and face ...... throbbing of the carotid and temporal arteries.... *(Peters 1853)*

A full-blown, plethoric appearance, as Peters describes, is distinctly uncommon, occurring in less than a tenth of cases of common migraine. Patients predisposed to red migraines often have a marked propensity to flush with anger or blush with embarrassment: facial erythema, we may say, is their "style".

A man of irascible temperament subject to common migraines since the age of 18, and bilious attacks and severe motion sickness in childhood. He has a beef-red-face, with tiny dilated arterioles in the nose and eyes. He flushes in his frequent rages, and indeed his face always seems to glow with a red smouldering fire which is the precise physiological counterpart of his chronic smouldering irritability. His face becomes crimson a few minutes before the onset of migraine headache, and remains flushed throughout the attack.

Such attacks would of course suggest remedies such as Belladonna, Sanguinaria and Sulphur and the bowel nosode Morgan.

Much more familiar is the picture of white migraine in which the face is pale, or even ashen, thin, drawn and haggard, while the eyes appear small, sunken, and ringed. The changes may be so marked as to suggest the picture of surgical shock. Intense pallor is always seen if there is severe nausea. On occasion, the face becomes flushed in the first few minutes of attack, and then abruptly pale, as if, in Peters' words, "all the blood passed suddenly from the head to the legs."

Remedies such as Lycopodium, Arsenicum, Nat. Mur. and Silicea are suggested and Veratrum which has paleness and collapse.

Oedema of the face and scalp may occur, either as isolated features in the context of a very general fluid-retention and, oedema may occur at the inception of the attack in some patients. In one such patient, observed at the inauguration of an attack, massive periorbital oedema developed on one side a few minutes before the onset of headache. More commonly, facial and scalp oedema develop after prolonged dilatation of extracranial vessels, and are associated, as Wolff and others have shown, with fluid transudation and sterile inflammation about the involved vessels. The oedematous skin is always tender and has a lowered pain threshold.

Ocular symptoms

It is almost always possible to detect changes in the appearance of the eyes during or before an attack of migraine headache, even though the patient himself may not volunteer any visual or ocular symptoms. There is usually some suffusion of small vessels in the globe, and in particularly severe attacks the eyes may become grossly bloodshot (this feature is characteristic in attacks of migrainous neuralgia). The eyes may appear moist (chemotic) from an increase in lachrymation — analogous to, and often synchronized with, the increases in salivation or bleary from an exudative inflammation of the vascular bed. Alternatively, the eyes may appear lustreless and sunken; a true exophthalmus may occur.

These changes in the eye ball, when severe may be associated with a variety of symptoms; itching and burning in the affected eye(s), painful sensitivity to light, and blurring of vision. Blurring of vision may be of incapacitating severity (blind headache) and one may find it impossible to visualize the retinal vessels with any clarity at such times, due to the exudative thickening of the cornea.

With Gelsemium heavy eyes are noted, Belladonna has injected eyes, and Nux too. Increased lachrymation is associated with Chelidonium, Rhus, Spigelia.

Nasal Symptoms

Descriptions of migraine rarely pay much attention to nasal symptoms although careful questioning of patients will reveal that at least a quarter of them develop some "stuffiness" of the nose in the course of an attack. Examination at this time will show enlarged and purple turkinates. Such symptoms and findings, when they are present, may mislead both patient and physicians into making a diagnosis of "sinus" or "allergic" headache.

Another nasal symptom, which may come either towards the beginning or at the resolution of the attack, is a profuse catarrhal secretion.

Abdominal symptoms and abnormal bowel action

About one-tenth of adults who suffer from common migraine complain of abdominal pain or abdominal bowel action during the course of the attack. The proportion is notably higher in younger patients, and the abdominal symptoms described here in a way constitute the predominant or only symptoms in so-called "abdominal migraines". Two types of abdominal pain are described with some frequency: the first is an intense, steady, boring "neuralgic" type of pain usually felt in the upper abdomen and sometimes radiating to the back it may mimic the pain of a perforated ulcer cholecystatis or pancreatitis. Somewhat colicky abdominal pain, often referred to the right lower quadrant and not infrequently taken for appendicitis.

Abdominal distension, visceral silence and constipation tend to occur in the prodromal or earlier portions of a migraine and contrast studies performed at this stage have confirmed that there is stasis and dilatation throughout the entire gastro-intestinal tract. This is succeeded in the later or closing portions of the attack by increased peristaltic activity thoughout the gut, clinically manifest as colicky pain, diarrhoea, gastric regurgitation.

Abdominal pains associated with headache are reviewed later, but Colocynth, Cina and Veratrum album, Aloes and Cocculus are some of the lesser-known remedies that can be used.

Lethargy and drowsiness

Although many patients, especially indomitable and obsessional ones, make no concessions to a migraine and insist on driving themselves the rough and usual round of work and play, a degree of listlessness and a desire for rest are characteristic of all severe common migraines. A vascular headache exquisitely sensitive to motion of the head may in itself enforce inactivity, but one cannot accept this as the only, or even the chief mechanism at work. Many patients feel weak during an attack and exhibit diminished tone of skeletal muscles. Many are dejected and seek reclusion and passivity. Many are drowsy.

It is important to distinguish this drowsiness from the comparatively natural and graceful sleep which, in a large proportion of cases, terminates and sometimes shortcuts the paroxysm. It is on the contrary of a most uncomfortable and oppressive character, sometimes verging on coma:

Livering compares this drowsiness with the altered states of consciousness which may sometimes precede an asthmatic attack, citing the following introspective and oppressive character, sometimes verging on coma.

"Symptoms of an approaching fit begin to appear at 4 PM. The principal symptoms were fullness in the head, dullness and heaviness of the eyes, and disagreeable drowsiness. The drowsiness increased so much that I spent great part of the evening in a succession of "trauces" as I call them. This horrid drowisness generally prevents one from being sensible of the approach of a fit till it has commenced."

Sometimes the drowsiness may precede other symptoms by minutes or hours, while at other times it presents itself *pari passu* with the headache and other symptoms. Repeated yawning is a characterstic feature of these lethargic states, presumably an attempted arousal mechanism, to stave off the torpor. Migrainous drowisness is not only "irresistible", glutinous and unpleasantly toned, but tends to be charged with peculiarly vivid, atrocious and incoherent dreams, a state verging on delirium. It is best, therefore, not to yield to it. Some patients do, however, discover that a brief deep sleep near the commencement of a migraine may prevent its subsequent evolution.

The duration of such curative sleep may be very brief. Living cites the case of a grader with typical abdominal migraines; this patient was able to shorten the development of full-blown attack if he could lie down under a tree and secure ten minutes' sleep at its inception.

Headaches associated with drowsiness call to mind *Gelsemium* and lesser known *Indium, Ailanthus, Leptandra* and *Chelidonium.*

Dizziness, vertigo, faintness and syncope

The vertigo must be considered quite exceptional in the course of common migraine, although it is often experienced in a migraine aura or classical migraine. Milder states of "lightheadedness" occur with notable frequency. Selby and Lauce (1960) in a clinical study of 500 patients with migraines of all types, found that "some 72% complained of a sensation of dizziness, lightheadedness and unsteadiness....". They further observed that "sixty patients out of 396 had lost consciousness in association with attacks of headaches.

The possible causes of such symptoms may, of course, be multiple, and will include automatic reactions to pain and nausea, vasomotor collapse, prostration due to fluid loss or exhaustion, muscular weakness and adynamia, etc; in addition to the action of direct central mechanisms inhabiting the level of consciousness.

Alterations of fluid balance

A number of migraine patients complain of increased weight, or tightness of clothes, rings, belts, shoes, etc., in association with their attacks. These symptoms have been submitted to precise experimental investigation by Wolff. Some weight-gain preceded the headache stage in more than a third of the patients he studied; since, however, the headache could not be influenced either by experimental diuresis or hydration, Wolff concluded that "weight gain and widespread fluid retention are concomitant but not causally related to headache".

During the period of water retention, urine is diminished in output and highly concentrated. The retained fluid is discharged through a profuse diuresis, sometimes associated with other secretory activities, as the migraine attack resolves.

A man who has had migraine headache for 4 years, knows the previous day he is about to suffer the bout. For, the day before he experiences compulsive eating and drinking. He retains fluids and puts on weight and when the headache is on the verge of breaking, he passes urine profusely. The day before he also suffers anxiety in his stomach, bounding heart and awful depression. Spigelia and Pulsatilla were two remedies this man benefited by. Gelsemium is often also associated with this symptom. Ignatia and Sanguinaria have polyuric symptoms alongside a headache.

Fever

Many patients may complain that they feel feverish during the course of a common migraine and they may indeed demonstrate flushing of the face, coldness and cyanosis of the extremities, shivering, sweating and alternating feeling of heat and cold preceding or accompanying the onset of headache.

These symptoms are not necessarily accompanied by fever, although the latter may be present, and are of considerable severity, specially in youthful patients.

Minor symptoms and signs

Contraction of one pupil, ptosis and exophthalmos

(Horner's syndrome) may produce a striking asymmetry in cases of unilateral migraine. There is no consistency, however, concerning pupillary size. In the earlier stages of an attack, or if pain is very intense, the pupils may be enlarged; later in an attack, or if nausea, lethargy, collapse, etc., dominate the picture, small pupils will be seen. The same consideration apply to pulse-rate: an initial tachycardia is likely to be followed by a protracted bradycardia, the latter sometimes associated with significant hypotension and postural faintness or syncope. Observant patients may comment on such changes of pulse and pupil during their worst attacks.

There is no end to the number of odd, miscellaneous alternations of physiological function which may occur as a result of migraine, a complete listing of these would provide a fascinating catalogue of curiora. It will suffice, however, to make brief reference to the occurrence of widespread vascular changes and occasional trophic changes associated with migraines.

Flushing of the entire body has been reported and the appearance of spontaneous ecchymoses of the limbs. The literature makes reference to whitening and loss of scalp hair though rarely noted.

Organic Irritability

.... The patient could not bear anything to touch his head and the least sight or sound, even the ticking of his watch was insupportable." *(Tissot. 1778)*

Irritability and photophobia are exceedingly common in the course of migraine attacks and have been adopted, by Wolff and others, as pathognomonic features aiding the diagnosis.

We are concerned with two types of irritability as accompaniments of the migraine state. The first is an aspect of the mood-change and defensive seclusion which may be so prominent in the behaviour and social posture of many migraine patients. The second type of irritability arises from a diffuse sensory excitation and excitability, so great that it may render all sensory stimuli intolerable as the old words of Tissot remind us. In particular, migraine patients are prone to photophobia, an intense discomfort, both local and general, provoked by light, and an avoidance of light which may become the most obvious external characteristic of the entire attack. Some of this photophobia is on the basis of conjunctival hyperaemia and inflammation, as described earlier and is associated with burning and smarting of the eyes. But a major cause of photophobia is a central irritability and sensory arousal.

An exaggeration and intolerance of sounds — photophobia — is equally characateristic of the severe attack; distant sounds, the noise of traffic, or the dripping of the top, may appear unbearably loud and provoke the patient to fury.

Very characteristic of this state is an exaggeration and often a perversion of the sense of smell; delicate perfumes appear to stink and may elicit an overwhelming reaction of nausea. Similarly with the sense of taste the blandest foods acquiring intense and often disgusting flavors.

It is important to note that sensory excitability of this type may precede the onset of headache, and in general, is characteristic of the early portions of the migraine attack. it is often followed by a state of sensory inhibition or indifference for the remainder of the attack. The alternation of sensations and sensory threshold which occur in common migraine, however distressing to the patient are very mild in comparison to the intense hallucinations and perversions of sensation which are characteristic of migraine aura and classical migraine.

Irritability and sensitivity are common symptoms in migraine and are not necessarily ultimate pointers to a remedy, but Nux, Bryonia, Chamomilla, Ignatia, Anacardium, and Belldonna as associated.

Mood Changes

Profound affective changes may occur during and only during a migraine attack, changes which are particularly startling in patients of normally equable temperament. Moreover, it will become clear that such mood changes are not simply reactions to pain, nausea, etc. but are themselves primary symptoms proceeding concurrently with the many other symptoms of the attack. Very profound mood-changes may also occur before and after the bulk of the attack, and as such will be considered later. The most important emotional colourings during the clinically recognised portion of a common migraine are states of anxious and irritable hyperactivity in the early portions of the attack, and states of apathy and depression in the bulk of the attack.

The common picture of anxious irritability has laready been sketched in the preceding section. The patient is restless and agitated; if confined to his bed, he will move about constantly, rearranging the bedclothes, finding no position of comfort; he will tolerate neither sensory nor social intrusions. His irascibility may be extreme. Such states are exacerbated if the patient continues to drive himself through his habitual routine of work, and their exacerbation, by a vicious circle, is likely to provoke a further increase in other symptoms of the attack.

Very different is the picture presented in the fully established or protracted attack. Here the physical and emotional posture is characterized by accepted suffering, dejection and passivity. Such patients unless compelled to act otherwise by internal or external factors, withdraw or regress into illness, solitude and seclusion. The emotional depression at such time is very real, often serious and occasionally suicidal. The following account is taken from an 18th century description:

"From the first perception of uneasiness in the stomach, the spirits begin to flag. They grow more and more depressed, until, cheerful thoughts and feelings fly away; and the patient conceives himself the most wretched of human beings and feels as if he were never to be otherwise."

The old description brings out the true depressive quality — the sense of utter hopelessness and permanence of misery — a reaction which is clearly far in excess of a realistic response to a shortlived benign attack of which the patient has had innumerable experiences.

Feelings of depression will be associated with feelings of anger and resentment, and in the severest migraines there may exist a very ugly mixture of despair, fury and loathing of everything and everyone not excluding the self. Such states of enraged hopelessness may be intolerable both for the patient and his family and should not be under-rated. The anger remedies include Nux vomica, Ignatia and Chamomilla.

Symptom-Constellations in Common Migraine

There have now been listed the major symptoms of a

common migraine as if these are unrelated to one another and occur at random. Certain groups of symptoms tend, however to occur with some consistency. The severe vascular headache usually occurs in association with other evidences of dilatation in extracranial vessels; suffusion and chemosis of the eyes, vascular engorgement within the nose, facial flushing etc. In other patients, gastro-intestinal symptoms form a coherent phalanx: gastric and intestinal distension, abdominal pains followed by diarrhoea and vomiting. A "shock" picture is seen in severe "white" migraines, constituted by pallor, coldness of the extremities, profuse cold-sweating, chilliness, shivering, slowness and feebleness of the pulse and postural hypotension; this picture is frequently seen in association with very severe nausea, but may occur when nausea is not prominent.

These three types are but three of many variants but in a later section an attempt will be made to relate these types to Paterson's bowel nosodes. There is a fairly obvious physiological linkage of symptoms in a particular symptom-picture, but in Homoeopathy one is looking for more than this, one is looking for the homoeopathic symptom-picture.

The sequence of a common migraine

As generally understood and described, a common migraine is constituted by vascular headache, nausea, increased splanchnic activity (vomiting, diarrhoea, etc.), increased glandular activity (salivation, lachrymation, etc.) muscular weakness and atonia, drowsiness and depression. We will find, however, that migraine neither starts nor ends with these symptoms and states which are clinically and physiologically the reverse of these.

We may speak of premonitory or prodromal symptoms, while recognizing that these pass, insensibly, into the earlier phases of the attack proper. Some of these prodromal or early symptoms are local, some systemic, some are physical and others are emotional. Among the commoner physical prodromes we must include states of water retention and thirst, states of visceral dilatation and constipation, states of muscular tension and sometimes hypertension. Among the emotional symptoms we must recognise states of hunger, restless, hyperactivity, insomnia, vigilance and emotional arousal which may have either an anxious or euphoric colouring. A sufferer from severe common migraines would speak of feeling "dangerously well" the day before his attacks. Such states, when they are acute and extreme, may achieve an almost maniacal intensity. Milder forms of this are quite common.

A woman who had lead a hard life, having spent most of her childhood at an orphanage, would suffer migraine headaches mostly at a weekend. But the day before her headache she would walk with 'real bounce in her step" and feel doubly well.

The resolution of a common migraine or indeed of any variety of migraine attack, may proceed in three ways, as has been recognised since the 17th century. It may, in its natural course, exhaust itself and end in sleep. The post-migrainous sleep is long, deep and refreshing, like a post epileptic sleep. Secondly, it may resolve by "lysis", a gradual abatement of the suffering accompanied by one or more secretory activities. As Calwell wrote, almost 150 years ago:

"Vomiting sometimes terminates a migraine. An abundant flow of tears does the same, or an abundant secretion of urine. Sometimes hemicrania is terminated by an abundant perspiration from the feet, hands, half of the face or by a nose bleeding, a spontaneous arterial haemorrhage, or a mucous flux from the nose."

The third mode of resolution of a migraine is by crisis — a sudden accession of physical or mental activity, which brings the attack to an end within minutes.

There has already been intimated an analogy between migraine and sleep, and this analogy is dramatized by the sense of extreme refreshment, and almost of rebirth, which may follow a severe but compact attack. Such states do not represent a mere restoration to the pre-migraine condition, but a swing in the direction of arousal, a rebound after the migrainous trough. In the words of Living : "........ (the patient) awakes a different being". Rebound euphoria and refreshment is particularly common after severe menstrual migraines. It is least in evidence after a protracted attack with vomiting fail to "recharge" the patient, and necessitate a period of convalescence.

Migraine Equivalents

Consideration of the many symptoms which may compose a common migraine has shown us that the term cannot be identified with any one symptom. A migraine is an aggregate of innumerable components and its structure is composite. The emphasis of the components is extremely variable within the framework of a general pattern. Headache may be the cardinal symptom; it may even be entirely absent. We use the term "migraine equivalent" to denote symptom complexes which possess the generic features of migraine but lack of specific headache component.

The concentrated experience of working with migraine patients must convince the physician, whatever his previous beliefs that many patients do suffer repeated, discrete, paroxysmal attacks of abdominal pain, chest pain, fever, etc., which fulfil every clinical criterion of migraine save for the presence of headache. Some of these variations are here reviewed:

Cyclic vomiting and bilious attacks

Frequency and severity of nausea is a component of juvenile migraines. Frequently, it forms the cardinal symptoms of a migraine reaction, and as such is often signified with the term "bilious attack". Selby and Lance provide the following figures from their large series:

"......Of 198 cases (of migraine) 31% recalled frequently occurring bilious attacks; of a further 139 patients,59% have a history of some bilious attacks or severe motion sickness during their early years".

Severe nausea is always accompanied by multiple autonomic symptoms — pallor, shivering, diaphoresis, etc.

A majority of attacks are put down to dietary indiscretion in childhood and in adult life ascribed to "gastric flu" or gall-bladder pathology, according to the persuation of the physician.

Such attacks may persist throughout life, or may undergo a gradual or sudden transition to the "adult form" — common migraine. The following case-history, provided by Vahlquist and Hackzell (1949), illustrates the genesis and evolution of such attacks in a young patient:

"..... When he was 10 months old he was badly frightened by an air-raid siren and after this had abnormal fear-reactions.... The first typical attack occurred at the age of one year. He suddenly turned pale, and later had an attack of violent vomiting. During the next two years he had several attacks a week always of the same type.... when he was about three, he began to complain of a pain in his head during the attacks. They generally ended in a heavy sleep".

Abdominal migraine

The symptoms in any type of migraine are multiple and the division between "bilious attacks" and "abdominal migraines is an interesting one". A case will be made in this thesis for differentiating biliousness from abdominal migraine on the basis that the former is covered by Paterson's Morgan nosode and the latter by Paterson's Protens nosode. The former shows a congested liverish bilious nature, the latter a picture of cramp and explosiveness. The dominant feature in the latter is epigastric pain of cramping character and great severity, accompanied by a variety of further automatic symptoms. The following incisive description is provided in Living's monograph:

"When about 16 years old, enjoying otherwise excellent health, I began to suffer from periodic attacks of severe pain in the stomach...... The seizure would commence at any hour and I was never able to discover any cause for it, for it was preceded by no dyspeptic symptoms or disordered bowels ...... The pain began with a deep, ill-defined uneasiness in the epigastrium. This steadily increased in intensity during the next two or three hours and then declined. When at its height the pain was very intolerable and sickening-it had no griping quality whatever. It was always accompanied by chilliness, cold extremities, a remarkably slow pulse and a sense of nausea — when the pain began to decline there was generally a feeling of movement in the bowels .... The paroxysm left very considerable tenderness of the affected region, which took a day or two to clear off, but there was no tenderness at the time".

Some years later, this particular patient ceased to have his abdominal attacks but developed instead attacks of classical migraine coming at similar intervals of three to four weeks.

The remedies for abdominal migraine would fall into the Protens category and would include, *Nat.mur.*, *Cuprum*, *Secale* and *Sepia*.

Here is a case of abdominal migraine, which was not cured by treatment. A 66 year old woman had migraines at the age of 50. It presented itself at first as follows: The pain would start on the left side of her abdomen and move to a burning pain and would later develop a feeling as if there was a blockage. The burning pain would spread all over the abdomen and then up the spine. Later on the pains became associated with sinus congestion, lachrymation, pain in the neck and later on still a typical migraine headahce. But the headache was not associated at first with these attacks. Arsenicum Alb. gave a temporary relief, but Homoeopathy did not help in the long term.

Precordial Migraine

The term "precordial migraine" (pectoralgic or pseudo-anginal migraine) denotes the occurrence of chest pain as a major constituent of a common or classical migraine or its occurrence as a periodic, paroxysmal symptom with migrainous rather than anginal qualities and antecedents.

The presentation and diagnosis of such attacks has been very finely considered by Fitg-Hugh (1940). Both Peterson's nosodes of Dys. Co and Protens are relevant in the precordial migraine picture, but if cramp is predominant a Protens remedy is indicated.

Periodic Sleep and Trance-states

The drowsiness which often accompanies or precedes a severe common migraine is occasionally abstracted as a symptom in its own right and may then constitute the sole expression of the migrainous tendency. The following case illustrates the "transformation" of common migraine to a sleep equivalent.

A woman started migraine attacks after first pregnancy with classical stonata, paraesthesial in half of the face and half of the tongue followed by a left sided headache that lasted 24 hours. Nausea, vomiting, loss of vision and distorted vision were common. She was greatly helped at this time by Homoeopathy and was completely free of headache for several years.

Lycopodium 10M and Bidor were the two remedies that secured this cure. Mentally she presented a conscientious, ambitious, introspective and intellectual woman. She easily tired at evening time. At the menopause, however, she started experiencing dreamy turns. She would talk to people then dream off. Dreamy turns would come while under pressure and she would act as if in a trance. She would dread the night following one of these attacks on account of the nightmares experienced. Homoeopathic treatment helped these greatly and they became less frequent. A combination of remedies was tried in succession : *Sulphur, Silicea, Arg.nit., Hyoscyamus* and, of course, *Nux moschata,* but the improvement was never marked enough to single out one remedy as curative. Bidor was frequently prescribed.

Menstrual Syndromes

A large minority of women experience marked affective and autonomic disturbances about the time of mestruation. Greene has estimated that "about 20 women in every 100 suffer sometimes from premenstrual migraine", and if we include under this heading autonomic and affective disturbance not accompanied by headache the figure must be substantially higher than this. Indeed, we may say that the menstrual cycle is always associated with some degree of physiological disturbance, even though this may pass unobserved by the patient. The disturbance tends to be in the direction of psycho-physiological arousal prior to menses, and "let down" followed by rebound after the menses.

The arousal period may be characterized by "tension", anxiety, hyperactivity, insomnia, fluid retention, thirst, constipation, abdominal distention, etc., and, more rarely asthma, psychosis, or epilepsy. The "let-down", period or "derousal" may be manifest as lassitude, depression, vascular headache, visceral hyperactivity, pallor, sweating, etc. In short, virtually all the symptoms of migraine, as they have been described thus far, may be condensed into the biological turmoil surrounding menstruation.

Of particular relevance in the present context is the frequent alternation, during the life-history of a single patient, of different formats of menstrual syndrome, with the emphasis on vascular headache at one time, at another on intestinal cramping, etc. The following case-history illustrates a sudden "transformation" between two types of menstrual migraine.

A woman had experienced severe abdominal (probably intestinal) cramping at the menstrual period between the ages of 17 and 30. She suddenly ceased to experience these symptoms at that age, but suffered in their place, typical premenstrual migraine headaches.

Other patients may suffer severe menstrual syndromes for several years, lose these to acquire frequent attacks of paroxysmal headache or abdominal pain related to the menstrual periods, finally reverting to the original pattern of menstrual disturbance. But there are many ways in which migraine headaches can inter-relate with the menstrual periods, as various in fact as woman herself and her complex psychology. The menopause can relieve migraine to worsen it, as can hysterectomy.

A woman had suffered headaches all her life which had started with her periods. They were not severe until middle age and were not associated with vomiting. She openly admitted to severe frustration due to having no outlet for her sexual energies. She was talkative, emotional and verged on the hysterical. She was recentful at life generally. She underwent a hysterectomy at the age of 47 for menorrhagia.

Ten years later the headaches became really severe and migrainous. She would suffer "knots in her abdomen " from tension and tachycardia. *Natrum Mur.* 10 M and *Bidor* were given to this patient with great relief experienced.

A 56- year-old woman suffered headaches since 7 years of age. Marriage eased the situation and lessened the frequency of the headaches, but they returned in force at the age of 50. At that time she was experiencing heavy periods with bleeding every three weeks and a hysterectomy was performed. After the operation the headaches were still severe and it was not until this patient was given relaxation thereapy in art classes and neck manipulation that true relief was experienced. She was a constant worrier and ambitious in her drives. From an early age she had felt the need to better her sisters who were always held upto her as an example. *Sepia 200* and *Pulsatilla 30*, together with *Lachesis 200* were remedies that gave relief.

In some cases definite relief from migraine is experienced at the menopause. A woman had suffered migraines on and off for ten years. The headache would occur just before the periods and were associated with severe premenstrual tension. She suffered severe blinding headaches that would centre on the top of her head. her emotional life at home was far from happy. There was a long standing feud with the daughter and the patient experienced anger and frustration in this relationship. She was impulsive, sympathetic and sensitive. She was prone to tears easily. Since her periods stopped 4 years previously she had been much improved. Menodoron had been prescribed in drop form with success and *Sulphur 30* and *Sepia 30* had both given good therapeutic results.

Summary

An attempt has been made in the preceding pages to give an idea of the complexity of migriane. There is not one migraine, there are many. Migriane is dynamic happening and intimately related to the patient's psychology, constittution, social evnvironment and place in life. The form that migraine takes relies to a large extent on the physique and make up of the individual. This is perhaps where Homoeopathy comes into its own, where the homoeopathic constitution plays a part. But again care should be taken not to rigidly set individuals into certain categories and there leave them. Migraine is an expression of need in the individual. It is a release force in itself and should be seen as such. Probably many remedies can benefit the same patient at different times both during his attacks and during his whole life experience of migraines. In the next section an attempt is made to set the migraine pattern against the large-scale back-drop of biology, psychology and energy release. An attempt is made to see the disease more in its totality and highlight its volatile nature. By so doing the importance of Paterson's bowel nosodes and the concepts he formed of the different nosode "types" comes early in to its own. The nosodes are seen as a valuable aid to homoeopathic treatment.

The Structure of Migraine

Let us examine in closer detail the structure of migraine. The sequence of a typical migraine might be as follows:-

1.   The initial excitement or excitation of an attack, emotionally experienced as rage, elation etc, and in the sense nervous system as sensory hyperacusis,

sensitivity to stimuli scintillating scotomata, paraestheiae, etc, accompanied by Vaso-constriction.

2. State of engorgement in the early stages, characterized by visceral distention and stasis, vascular dilations, faecal retention, fluid retention, muscular tension, etc, and concurrently with these symptoms feelings of emotional tension, anxiety, restlessness, irritability etc.

3. A state of prostration characterized by apathy, depression and retreat, while its physical concomitants are nausea, malaise, drowsiness, faintness, muscular slackness, and weakness.

4. A state of recovery or resolution, which may be achieved abruptly (crisis) or gradually (lysis). In the case of the former, there may occur a violent visceral ejaculation (vomiting or even sneezing); in the case of the latter a variety of secretory activities (diuresis, diaphoresis, involuntary weeping etc.) all representing a catharsis of a certain emotional state.

5. A stage of rebound (if the attack has been brief and compact) accompanied by euphoria and renewed energy. If one could telescope these phenomena for the sake of clarification one could say there is a stage of acute excitation of the sense nervous system, and related automatic system, followed by a phase of inhibition. The relationship here between epilepsy and migraine is seen to be close. It is important to note, too, that migraine is no more a suspension of physical and mental activities than sleeping. It is charged, on the contrary, with activities of an inward

private kind. Inhibition at one level releases excitations at other levels. The diminution of motor activity and external relationship during a migraine is matched by a great increase in internal activities, vegetative symptoms and their attendant effects - a paradoxical combination of inner violence and outer detachment.

Liveing in the 19th century in his clearly written doctrine on migraine distinguishes the notion of nerve force or energy in the nervous system from accumulation of any one substance. The biochemical theories of our time mislead in that they draw one away from observing the attack of migraine as a general phenomenon and would tend to concentrate one's attention on one particular chemical reaction going on at one particular level of the brain. Chemical reactions are concomitant phemomena, not casual ones.

Liveing writes: ".....a gradually increasing instability of equilibrium in the nervous parts; when this reaches a certain point, the balance of forces is liable to be upset and the train of paroxysmal phenomena determined by causes in themselves totally inadequate to produce such effects.

He comes to this conclusion from a consideration of the enormous number of factors of different kinds which can precipitate an attack: "..... the impression may come from without, and be of the nature of an irritation of some peripheral nerve, visceral, muscular, or cutaneous; or it may reach the centres through the circulation ...... or it may descend from the higher centres of physical activities...."

So many exciting factors, yet the effect is the same; in every case the nervous system responds with a migraine. Therefore, the migraine is implicit in the cerebral repertoire. Its structure is, as it were profound.

Liveing recognizes that a migraine can act as a consummatory discharge, following and terminating the build up of a tension; thus he compares it with a sneeze, a voracious meal or an orgasm. Indeed, these discharges may be "equivalent", and are thus liable to metamorphoses among themselves; he instances the ability of fit or sneezing suddenly to terminate, or replace a migraine; or the apprehension of sudden danger terminating an intense seasickness; sexual excitement provoking an asthma; or ticking an epilepsy.

The last thirty years have witnessed an intensive search for vascular, chemical and electrical disturbances occurring in relation to migraine attacks, and a proliferation of theories postulating physical abnormalities as essential fundamental mechanism in causation of attacks. These theories at best, however, are but partial answers, can never explain the whole migraine phenomenon and are self limiting. Vaso-constriction, vaso-dilation and release of serotonin are chemical results and not primary causes in themselves.

The Psychology of Migraine

Migraine is a remarkably primitive reaction including massive alterations of vegetative activity and of general activity and behaviour. We have considered migraine thus far, as the symptoms of which a patient may complain and at this level, obviously, we can derive no information from animals which may suffer but cannot express, complaints. If we are to form any picture of the biological role of migraine, and of its homologous and analogous in the animal world, we must instead concern overselves with the behaviour of the migraine patient and the circumstances to which the behaviour has relevance.

Let us then construct a picture of migrainous behaviour. As the symptoms mount, the patient will go to his room and lie down, he will have the blinds drawn and the children hushed; he will tolerate no intrusions. The intensity of his symptoms will drive other thoughts from his mind; he may be sunk, if the attack is very severe, in a leaden, stuporous daze. He pulls the blanket over his head, excluding the outer world, and enveloping himself in the inner world of his symptoms. He says to the world: "Go away. Leave me alone. This is my migraine. Let me suffer in peace." At length, perhaps, he falls asleep. And when he wakes, it is all over, the migraine is done, its work is accomplished; there may be a post migrainous surge of energy, almost literally a re-animation. The essential therms of the attack are these: retreat from the outer world, regression, and finally, recuperation.

In some-what less form at terms, the migraine reaction tends to be characterized by passivity, stillness and immobilization; commerce with the outer world is minimal, while inner activities - particularly of secretory and expulsive type - are minimal. It is in these general terms that we may perceive the primary adaptive function of a migraine and in these terms that we may seek for parallel reactions both in the human and animal world.

It is a protective reflex that we envisage the primary role of migraine, as withdrawal of the whole body from "the operation of noxious or endangering stimulus", in short as a particular form of reaction to threat concurrent with the role, and perhaps inseparable function, both of which would seem to be of particular relevance when the "harmful agent is felt or symbolised as a harmful or hateful emotional situation.

"Response to threat, in the animal world may take either or both of two fundamentally different forms. The form which is most familiar, and which springs immediately to mind is the use of an active physical response, the fight-flight response, with its emotional correlates of rage or terror.

The fight-flight reaction is dramatic in the extreme, but represents only half of biological reality. The other half is no less dramatic, but it is dramatic in contrary style. Its characteristics are those of passivity and immobilization in response to threat. The antitheses between these two styles of reaction was memorably described by Darwin in his comparison of active fear (terror) and passive fear (dread). In the former, says Darwin, there is "the sudden and uncontrollable tendency to headlong flight." The picture of passive fear as Darwin portrays it, is one of passivity and prostration, allied with increased splanchnic and glandular activity (".... a strong tendency to yawn ..... death like pallor ..... beads of sweat stand out of the skin. All the muscles of the body are relaxed. Utter prostration soon follows. The intestines are affected. The sphincter muscles cease to act, and no longer retain the contents of the body..."). The general attitude is one of cringing, cowering and sinking. If the passive reaction is more acute, there may be abrupt loss of postural tone or of consciousness. If the passive reaction is more protracted, the physiological changes are less dramatic, but still in the same direction. We find throughout the animal world a repertoire of passive reactions at least as important, and considerably more variable, than the active responses to threat. All of them are characterized by immobilization (with some inhibition of postural tone and arousal), usually in conjunction with increased secretory and splanchnic activity. A handful of examples will suffice. A fearful dog (specially if it belongs to Pavlov's weak inhibitory type) cowers, and may vomit and be incontinent of faeces; the hedgehog responds to threat by curling up. The frightened horse may "freeze" and break into a cold sweat; the threatened skunk freeze and secretes profusely from modified sweat-glands (here the secretory response has assumed an offensive function); the menaced chameleon freezes and changes colour to mimic the environment through another variant of internal secretion. It is clear that the passive response to threat has been utilized, from the start of life, as biological alternative to active reactions. The passive reaction, indeed, is frequently superior to the active response in terms of survival value. Where the aroused animal forces (or flees) danger and threat, the inhibitory reaction enables it to avert these, to become, one way or another, less accessible to danger.

The development of large social units and cultural repressions inseparable from this, have doubtless necessitated, as they have permitted, a far greater variety of vegetative retreats and protracted passive reactions than were previously possible. These psychosomatic reactions, along with neurotic defences and reactions, represent the only alternatives in situations where direct action is neither permissible nor possible. A complex world needs complex defences.

The circumstances the patient finds himself in are intimately related - usually - to the pattern of the migraine. It is well known for instance that migraines occur at weekends, and on the first day of holidays. These reactions can be grouped together as "slump reactions". There is a common characteristic of "let down" in the circumstance. Whether it is a missed meal, hot weather, exhaustion from hard work, or after a strenuous event, or a nocturnal migraine. In all these circumstances the person's defences are down and the movement of energies from metabolic regions into sense nervous regions takes place uninhibited. It is rather as if the terminals, positive and negative, can be connected, and resistance being lowered the current flows.

If one takes the analogy of electricity further, it helps to understand the phenomenon of arousal stimuli in migraine. Circumstances or stimuli which activate, arouse, annoy, or gangle the organism can trigger off a migraine reaction. They are enough to set the current flowing between the two poles. Light, noise, smells, climate, exercise, food, excitement and most important of all, violent emotion, can all precipitate an attack. The menstrual period is often related in the case of women to their migraine attacks and the psychological reasons for this relationship are often complex to unravel but significant. Hormonal and body fluid before a period and at the time of a period must impinge strongly upon the psyche of the patient. Premenstrual irritability, depression and mental disturbance is of common occurrence.

A woman suffered migraine headaches since the age of 40. They would come first before a period and would last 24 hours. She would be unable to read as her eyes would be out of focus. The headache was relieved by the period flow. Since her menopause she had been much better.

Pulsatilla and *Menodoron* both helped her attacks.

A woman suffered nausea, vomiting and severe pain in

the right eye with zig-zags in front of eyes and distorted vision since the age of 26. She was fastidious, sympathetic and unmarried. Her symptoms were made worse by the menopause. Sepia was the remedy that most helped her.

Referring to the circumstances and situations that surround migraine, sometimes a precipitating factor is obvious to see and sometimes not. It may not even be present as such. One may suppose that certain individuals have built into their system a certain nervous instability of the migrainous type. This then requires release at certain times independent of the environment. But such stimuli as noise, light, food and emotion are enough to spark off an attack of migraine.

Deeper than these superficialities lie the complexes that explain migraine in the psychological sphere and much work has been done on classifying and analysing these complexes. The outward experience of a migraine might well be that of "passive crisis" or "extreme helplessness", but the inward dynamics of the various forces of migraine are more complex. It is not necessary in such a work as this to detail the psychoanalytic arguments that have been developed relating to the migraine syndrome but mention can be made of the various categories that have been agreed upon. They help our understanding of the illness, and our homoeopathic prescribing.

Four basic types are recognised; the recuperative, the regressive, the encapsulative and the aggressive. Tolerance must be asked for following the introduction of such psychological "jargon". The types themselves however, are fairly obvious, though they often merge and overlap.

The first category - the recuperative - experience their migraine following prolonged physical or emotional activity. The notorious weekend attack. The phase or prostration may be profound and even stuporous. Euphoria and sense of awakening sometimes follows such attacks... Obsessive, conscientious and driving personalities can be subject to such attacks.

The second category - those who experience a regressive migraine, have taken their migraine a stage futher. Allied also to ennvironmental or emotional stress the migraine is both a "vegetative retreat" and a "cry for help". They are marked by pitiful suffering, dependency needs, a crippling of the personality. They are frequently found in illness prone individuals and hypochondriacs. They become an indulgence and are morbidly welcomed by the individual, unconsciously.

The third category - the encapsulative migraine, is also a variant upon the other two. There are a number of patients in whom periodic or sporadic migraines are experienced which seem to embed, enact and work through certain emotional conflicts. Menstrual migraines could well act by condensing the stresses of the month into a few days of concentrated illness. Treating such outlets in a superficial manner has been observed merely to displace the conflicts into another area, for instance, by spreading the neurotic energy into a general anxiety syndrome. The migraine could serve a purpose in binding or "encapsulating" the conflict.

In the aggressive migraine (if all migraines are not aggressive) there is a background of intensive chronic and repressed rage and hostility and the function of the migraine is to provide some expression of what cannot be expressed, or even acknowledged, directly. Such migraines often occur in family situations where relationships between individuals are intolerable to a degree. When the hostility is turned inward the attacks become self-punitive, masochistic, paranoid and self-destructive.

Examples of these various psychological aspects of migraines will be given in the following section on Nosodes. But it should be noted here that one particular case may show several aspects. All of us have aggressive tendencies which have to be repressed and all of us have work tensions which produce a need for recuperation. However, it is the way that these various aspects are blended in one particular case that makes the study worthwhile both from the point of view of psychology and, more important, in the case of this paper from the point of view of prescribing homoeopathic drugs.

Migraines can be said to arise as most disease can, from chronic repressed emotional needs. This would be perfectly acceptable psychological view point and reasonable one but it does not say very much. And if you call the emotional needs libido and say that migraine is an expression of repressed libido, you have said no more. A migraine should be seen as a function, as dissemination of energy through-out an unbalanced body system. When the individual migraine is observed in these various lights it becomes meaningful and then treatable. For as in all diseases there are many paths to healing, and the more the illness can be seen in depth and in true all round perspective, the more accessible it is to treatment.

Migraines fill a dramatic role in the emotional economy

of the individual. They perform a task of emotional equilibration, and as such are analogous to dreams, hysterical and neurotic symptoms, epilepsy and many other forms of dramatic human symptomotology. Migraines are both a physical event and an important inner event for the individual and in this latter aspects they are a form of symbolic draw into which the patient has transported important thoughts and feelings. Thus a rage migraine may be regarded as a complex but stereotyped reaction to rage, in patients who experience this. The earlier stages of such an attack (termed earlier phase of "engorgement") are likely to be characterised, emotionally, by irritability and angry tension, and physiologically by vascular and visceral dilation, fluid retention, oliguria, faecal retention, etc., the symptoms of a generalized sympathetic discharge. The patient is stuffed, impacted, and bloated with anger. The resolution of the attack may be preceded by crisis (brief forceful vomiting, sudden passage of flatus and faeces, sneezing, etc.,) or by lysis (diuresis, diaphoresis, epiphora, etc.). Thus the rage of such attacks is expressed in plethora, and discharged with a sudden visceral ejaculation or a slow secretory catharsis (analogous to weeping).

We must allow the possibility that not only may the entire migraine have meaning for the patient, but that certain individual symptoms of the attack may also be invested with specific symbolic importance, and further, that they may be susceptible to modification in accordance with this importance. We have seen that nausea and vomiting are cardinal symptoms of migraine; these could be said to signify disgust (feared, hated) of situation, person etc. The action of the bowels, initially determined by physiological needs and periodicities, ay be further determined, often overwhelmingly so, by the (unconscious) symbolic values attached to faeces and defaecation. Constipation and diarrhoea, wreathed with the variety of symbolic meanings, are among the commonest of functional disorders and also as we have seen, frequent and important parts of many migraines. Furmauski (1952) in an interesting character study of 100 migraine patients, has remarked on the frequency of "oral traits" and "anal traits" in this group, but has not attempted, regrettably, to determine whether there existed any correlation between these traits and the type of migraine experienced.

There presumably exist in every one of us particular physiological idiosyncracies, preferential pathways and mechanisms, which predispose a patient towards one migraine format rather than another. In certain rare and stereotyped forms of migraine such as hemiplegic migraine these formats are rigidly set. In others they are elastic and interchangeable, but physiology plays upon psychology and psychology profoundly affects physiology and the truth lies in the interaction between the two.

The Three - Part Body System

The interaction of these two fields-physiology and psychology becomes easier if we look at the human body as basically divided into three parts, striving continually to find a harmony and balance in their proportionate relationships. Life in all its dimensions is continually adjusting to achieve balance and nowhere is this more true than in the human body. The three areas are:

1. The head and sense nervous system

2. The chest, heart and shythunic system

3. The abdomen and metabolic system

The metabolic - abdominal area and the sense-nervous system represent two opposite poles of our human physiology.

The first is warm, continually renewing metabolizing filled with blood. The sense nervous system is bloodless by comparison, is not renewable and is static. It is rooted in the head, is the seat of thought and senses. The two polar opposites of fear and shame help us to realise these contrasts. Fear is the nerve process overstepping its normal limits. One can be petrified by fear. Shame is the blood process which can overwhelm us. One can be drowned in shame.

If there is a conflict between head and belly, resolution can take place by a passage of energy between the two and migraine is but a passage of energy from the belly to the head.

The metabolic energies have to be transmitted to the other two spheres and similarly nervous head energy in its right dimension must exert an effect upon the abdomen. But where unnaturally great energies are focussed or where there is inhibition then there is conflict and tension. Inhibition by the sense nervous system upon the free flowing metabolic energies can lead to a migraine reaction just as can too great a concentration of energy in the metabolic sphere *per se*. In the next section an attempt will be made to delineate certain forms of reaction that take place in these three spheres and relate these to the bowel nosodes of Paterson. This can give a very valuable clue to the appropriate homoeopathic remedy. Fear, anxiety and stress build up inhibitory barriers to free flowing energy patterns and are prescursors of disease.

The genesis of a migraine attack is often, as will be shown later, related to circumstances and situations. Frustration of the free flow of energies in a relaxed and harmonious way round the body leads to a build up in tension within the body. The trigger is released, the dam bursts and the metabolic energies flood the sense nervous system. An overwhelming assault *via* the automatic nervous system leads to such symptoms as have been enumerated, as various as human physiology will allow.

The various symptom complexes can then be seen to be a natural occurrence. The metabolic and dynamic causes are basically the same, the final outlet chosen may vary.

The differences between abdominal, precordial, febrile affective and other forms of migraine are not so significant after all. The human body can transmute one form of attack into another with ease. It would not be absurd to talk of paroxysmal asthma, angina and laryngospasm as being migraine equivalents. They could be filling a biological role analogous to that of migraine attacks. Heberden (1802) recorded the already established observation that "the hemicrania had ceased upon the coming of an asthma."

Asthma in this context could be looked upon as an envelopment of the shythemic sphere. If one supposes the inhibitions from the cortical nervous system are so strong as to prevent a migraine, one could postulate that the displaced energy from the metabolic areas meets the cortical inhibitions in the intermediate shythemic system, the gateway between the two, and produce an asthma.

Migraine must be seen to be a release phenomenon and if viewed as such it then becomes understandable. The manner of its release depends upon the make-up of the autonomic system, and the peculiarity of the psyche, in fact, the constitution of the individual. Here is where Homoeopathy plays its part.

Bowel Nosodes and Migraine

. The research work that has been done in Homoeopathy upon the bowel nosodes is inextricably linked with the name of John Paterson. He derived his nosodes and the mode of preparation from doctors Bach and Wheeler in the 1920's.

Doctors Bach and Wheeler in their work "Chronic Disease, a Working Hypothesis, describe how it was possible to isolate from the stool of patients suffering chronic disease certain non-lactose fermenting gram-negative bacilli. These bacilli when given back to the patient in the form of a Vaccine cured the diesease. They state:

"A point which we particularly wish to stress is that a non-lactose fermenting gram-negative bacillus in the faeces, whether it falls into a known variety or not, may be the cause of toxaemia, even though it may not give rise to obvious lesions."

Vaccine therapy principles warrant the belief that if disease symptoms disappear or are much ameliorated after the use of a vaccine made from a particular organism, then that organism counts at least for something in the production of the disease symptoms.

Referring to the bowel organism B. Coli Paterson introduces his study of the bowel nosodes as follows:-

"In nature where there is balance there is no disease

and the germ, in this case the B. Coli in the intestinal tract, performs a useful function. Where the intestinal mucosa is healthy the B. Coli is non-pathogenic. Any change in the host which affects the intestinal mucosa will upset the balance and will be followed by a change in the habit and the bio-chemistry of the B. Coli which may then be said to become pathogenic but it should be noted that the primary change, the 'disease', originated in the host, which compelled the bacillus to modify its habit in order to survive.

In 1936. Paterson presented a paper to the British Homoeopathic Society, which was published in their Journal of April 1936, under the title of "The Potentized Drug and its Action on the Bowel Flora." A brief summary of the findings is as follows:-

(A)   Non-lactose fermenting bacilli were isolated in 25 per cent of the stool specimens examined.

(B)   The appearance of non-lactose fermenting bacilli often followed and seemed to bear relationship to the previously administered homoeopathic remedey - the choice of the remedy being made according to" the law of similars and prepared by "potentization."

Paterson wrote of his findings as follows:-

"In the laboratory one observed an unexpected phenomenon, that from a patient who had previously yielded only B. Coli., there suddenly appeared a large percentage of non-lactose fermenting bacilli of a type which one associated with the pathogenic group of typhoid and paratyphoid."

"If one accepts the view, generally held, that the B. Coli of the intestinal tract is a harmless saprophyte and is non-pathogenic it must be concluded that, so far as the intestinal tract was concerned there was no evidence of disease in these patients during the first series of examinations. Now the patient's stool yielded a large percentage of presumably pathogenic organisms, and according to the accepted Pasteur and Koch theory, the patient was suffering from disease. Clinical investigations, however, revealed that the patient did not feel ill, but he experienced a sense of well being which he had attributed to the last medicine he had received. Since the non-lactose fermenting bacilli had appeared after the definite latent period of 10 to 14 days, following the administration of the remedy, it would seem that the homoeopathic potentized remedy had changed the bowel flora, and had caused the "disease". The pathogenic germ in this case was the result of vital action set up in the patient by the potentized remedy. The germ was not the cause of the disease.

"Is the "specific germ" the actual cause of disease, or is it the result of the action of the vital force (Dynamis) which characterised all living cells, in their resistance to disease? That is a question which I must ask you to consider and answer for yourselves in the light of the observations I have placed before you today. Meantime, it will be sufficient for the purpose of continuing the subject of this paper, if you agree that each germ is associated with its own peculiar symptom picture (disease) and that certain conclusions may be made from these clinical and laboratory observations and translated into the practice of medicine.

(A) The specific organism is related to the disease

(B) The specific orgamism is related to the homoeopathic remedy.

(C) The homoeopathic remedy is related to the disease."

(Paterson - 1950)

Paterson categorised the non-lactose fermenting organisms of the bowel into certain categories. they are as follows:-

Bacillus Morgan .... Gaertner.

Bacillus Morgan - Gaestuer .... Dys. Co.

Proteus .... Sycotic Co.

Bacillus No. 7 .... Mutabile.

A study has been made in this thesis of the relationship of four of these bowel nosodes and their symptom pictures to the migraine syndrome. The four nosodes most often associated seemingly with migraine are Bacillus Morgan, Morgan - Gaertuer, Proteus and Dys. Co.

Morgan.

Morgan is the bacillus most commonly found in faeces of the population and the keynote of the Morgan nosode is "congestion." The symptom picture is as follows:

Appearance :   Florid : dark more than fair

                                    Pale : either dark or fair.

Head : Congestive headaches, with flushed face; worse from hot atmosphere; thundery weather; excitement; travelling in bus or train.

Vertigo from high blood pressure.

Mentals : Introspective, anxious and apprehensive about state of health; irritability; avoids company but often shows mental anxiety if left alone.

Mental depression, often with suicidal tendency.

Digestive System : Congesting of gastric mucosa and liver; heartburn and a dirty tongue; bitter taste in mouth in the morning with accumulation of mucus causing gagging as soon as rises from bed. Congestion of liver: "bilious attacks" with severe headache which is finally relieved by vomiting large quantities of bile-stained vomitus. (A history of "bilious attacks," specially occurring at the menopause in women should lead one to consider the use of the nosode, Morgan (Bach).

Cholecystitis, gall stone; constipation, haemorrhoids pruritus ani.

Respiratory System : Congestion of nasal and bronchial membrane, especially in children, broncho - and lobar pneumonia. It is worth noticing, in view of the frequent use of the Sulpha drugs in the treatment of pneumonia, that sulphur is outstanding among the remedies associated with "Bacillus Morgan of the intestinal tract.

Genito-Urinary System: the congestive headache associated with the menstrual onset has already been mentioned, and this is often accompanied by ovarian pain (congestive dysmenorrhoea) or by the congestive flushings of menopause period Menorrhagia.

Circulation : Congestion and sluggish action is seen by the tendency to haemorrhages and varicose veins.

Fibrous Tissues : Chronic congestion around the joints causes arthritic conditions, usually affecting the phalangeal or knee joint regions.

Abdomen : Bilious attacks.
Epigastric pain or discomfort.
Tenderness epigastrium.
Pain right and left hypochondrium.
Pain right and left iliac fossae.

Pain liver and gall-bladder.
Tender liver and gall-bladder.
Gall-stones; confirmed by X-rays
or operation. Attacks of jaundice.

Bowels :

Constipation - present in 95 per
cent of present series. Pruritus
ani. Piles - bleeding; itching or
painful.

Skin :

It is here that the outstanding
action of the Bacillus Morgan group
organisms is to be found. Morgan
(Bach) is the nosode indicated
where there is congestion of the
skin with itching eruption, worse
from heat. The type of eruption
which characterises this can be
ascertained from a study of the
"provings" of well known skin
remedies found among the list of
remedies associated with the
Bacillus Morgan, e.g. **Sulphur,
Graphites, Petroleum, Psorinum,
Pulsatilla, Sepia, Calc carb, Kali
carb and Nux Vom.**

Proteus

Paterson states that Proteus will seldom have any
therapeutic reaction unless there are outstanding symptoms
in the case relative to the central or peripheral nervous
system and symptoms which appear with a degree of
suddenness. "Brain storm is the phrase which characterizes

this explosiveness and its applicability in the case on migraine is obvious.

The picture of Proteus is as follows:

Mentals :

Mental symptoms are prominent in the chemical proving and "Brain Storm" might be taken as the keynote to indicate this sudden and violent upset of the nervous system. Tense, irritable, depressed.

Outburst of violent temper, especially if opposed in any way; will throw any missile which is at hand, kick or strike; the child dejecting to parental control will be on the floor and kick and scream.

Emotional, hysteria, suggestive of the remedy Ignatia is also found in the proving of this B. Proteus preparation and convulsive and epileptiform seizures and meningismus in children during febrile attacks often responds to the action of the nosode Proteus (Bach). Further indication for the use of this nosode is disturbance of the peripheral nervous system evidenced by spasm of the peripheral circulation, e.g. "dead fingers"; intermittent claudication in the circulation of the lower limbs, anginal attacks due to spasm of the coronary capillaries.

There are two well-known diseases associated with capillary spasm where the nosode Proteus (Bach) has been found useful in treatment - Raynaud's disease, where there is spasm of the capillary circulation of extremities and Meniere's disease where spasm of the brain circulation results in vertigo attacks. Headache before menstrual period.

Digestive System :- It is important to note that any of the symptoms manifest in the digestive system are secondary to the action of the central nervous system. It is now being realised that prolonged nerve strain is a factor in the production of duodenal ulcer, and in the Proteus proving, this is also to be found. This is the type of case where there are no prodromal symptoms in the digestive system and the first sign is that of a haematemesis of melaena. These ulcers have a tendency to perforate, probably due to the innervation and interference with capillary circulation in that area. Acidity and heartburn do occur.

Neuro - muscular System :- As one might expect from the foregoing indications, cramp of muscles is a characterstic symptom and **Cuprum metallicum** is also found among the list of remedies. Pain in the chest, intermittent claudication. Angina.

Skin :- Angio neurotic oedema, which one associates with the remedy Apis mellifica is found in the proving of the B. Proteus preparation and also a tendency for the production of herpetic eruption at the muco-cutaneous margins.

Remedies associated are **Nat. mur., Cuprum, Secale, Kalimur., Mag mur.,** and **Calc mur.**

Paterson noted an increase in Proteus after the last war and associated it with nerve strain, continued over a long period.

Dys co.

This is the nosode prepared from B. Dystenteriae and the keynote for its use is nervous tension of a peculiar type and best described as "anticipatory." Since it is that sense of nerve tension which a student might feel immediately before facing his examiners, or a business man before attending an important engagement. The picture is as follows :-

Appearance : Thin

Fair hair, dark lashes, pink or white skin.

Dark hair, pale, good colour.

Mentals : Nervous tension, mental uneasiness in anticipation of some event;

hypersensitive to criticism; mental uneasiness among strangers; mental uneasiness shows itself by physical restlessness; cannot keep still, fidgets, dioreic movements of facial muscles, or limbs. Headache, frontal over the eyes, or in vertex, brought on by excitement; often occurs at regular time.

Periods of 7 to 14 days' cycle, associated with loose bowels.

More headache than vomiting in migraine.

Digestive System : Dysenterial has been shown to have selective action on the pylorus causing spasm and regurgitation of digested contents; dilation of stomach; wakened at 12 midnight to 1 A. M. with acute pain in stomach, relieved by vomiting of a large quantity of mucous material.

Food of fats, sweets, salt, milk. Indigested pain for years with distention and discomfort.

Heart burn.

Loose bowels.

Duodenal ulcer often calls for the use of nosode Dys. Co. (Bach)., but there must always be present also evidence of nervous tension, which always precedes the physical symptom and which the patient feels and refers to his" stomach and heart area". This is in contrast to the type of duodenal ulcer found associated with the B. Proteus, where the nerve tension is insidious in action, imperceived by the patient, and the physical condition-the ulcer- tends to come on as a "crisis" without previous warning.

Cardiovascular:	Functional disturbance of heart action, associated with nerve tension; palpitation before important events; anticipatory discomfort in the cardiac area.

These are the outstanding symptoms found in the clinical proving of the nosode Dys. Co (Bach), and they are found in each of the associated remedies, **Ars, alb, Arg.-nit; Kalmia.**

Morgan - Gaertner.

This is a variant of Bacillus Morgan, but a very important one. The picture is that of Lycopodium, the chief remedy of the group. Whereas Morgan has many skin symptoms, Morgan - Gaertner has strong emphasis on the urinary tract; renal stones, renal colic, cystitis, vulvo vaginitis are all covered well by this remedy. The mentals are akin to Morgan. Flatulence is the main symptom in the stomach syndrome, and respiratory symptoms are common.

Its picture is as follows:-

Appearance :	PALE faced (occasionaly florid), Dark haired.
Mentals :	Irritable, Quick tempered, impatient, tense.
	Nervous. Restless, weepy, depressed. Fear crowds.

Head :	Congestive headache. Flushed face.
Nose :	Nasal catarrh.
Mouth :	Bitter taste, bad taste.
Appetite :	Fond of sweets, salt and prefers hot food.
Stomach :	Flatulent indigestion; expressive eructation.
	Fullness in epigastrium.
Abdomen :	Flatulence, distension, Pain ileocaecal region.
	Pain gall-bladder, cholecystitis. Heartburn, constipation.
Genito-urinary System.	Renal colic, cystitis.

Associated remedy: **Lycopodium**.

It is dangerous to over-simplify and in the world of Homoeopathy we like to think that our remedies are chosen for each individual as a unique event. However we are all, if we are honest, simplifying and categorizing in our mind to a large degree, while we are choosing a remedy we have half a dozen" hot" remedies we know by heart and a dozen "cold" remedies. We have so many "tidy" remedies in our mind and favourite skin remedies, and so on.

It is possible to characterize various forms of migraine reaction and some of these have been outlined. One can define therefore certain categories of migraine observing the event as a dynamic happening, and observing the patient as a total individual. By fitting the two together one sees a form emerge that alongside our understanding of the nosodes, gives a clue to the indicated remedy.

We have so far analysed the migraine reaction in terms of psychology and also a flow of energies between three systems. To summarize briefly, a migraine reaction is seen as a flooding of the sense, nervous system by energies from the metabolic spheres. The autonomic nervous system is seen as the physiological "wiring" that enables this release of energy to occur while the psychology of the individual sets the tone, pattern and circumstances of the event.

If again the three part body system is visualized, the metabolic-abdominal region, the rhythmic chest system, and the head-sense-nervous system; in different people the energies are set at a different potential, they move in a different manner and are controlled by different stimuli.

Paterson spoke of Morgan as a live remedy and gave congestion as the keynote to the symptoms, indicating the importance of biliousness in the abdominal reaction. He spoke of "Cramp" on the other hand and "brain storm" as the key note of Proteus. The contrast between these two remedies can be nicely brought out in the study of the migraine reaction.

The following cases illustrate this :-

A woman had suffered migraines for years at first associated with her periods. She was round, fat, jolly, but suffered chronic indigestion and "liverishness". She had an appetite for most foods, but cream in abundance upset her. She had to rest after a meal or walk slowly or a bout of indigestion would occur. She tended to eat too quickly. She was prone to constipation. She stated that aggravation and disappointments in her life had made her ill. She was unmarried and suffered hypertension. Headaches were pressing and congestive. She loved people but easily got depressed and weepy. Often felt frustrated with life.

Pulsatilla and **Sulphur** are this lady's medicines, and she responded to the first. But Morgan is the bowel nosode. The liver is the organ of note.

Conclusions

It is not always obvious that a bowel nosode is indicated in any disease but where there are symptoms that point towards a nosode, the nosode should surely be given. In Homoeopathy today, the bowel nosodes are underused and undervalued. It has been the purpose of this thesis to analyse the total migraine reaction with a view to extending and improving our homoeopathic therapy with particular regard to the use of the bowel nosodes. Bach, Wheeler and Paterson were certain the chronic disease had to be treated differently to acute disease. It was not enough to give the indicated remedy or the "constitutional" remedy. What was needed was an approach to effectuate the chronic miasms that underlay disease. Until these were treated no effective cure would result.

Migraine is a syndrome that has certain dynamic patterns of reaction built into its physiology. It has been attempted in this thesis to break these down and analyse them so making the task of choosing a bowel nosode that much easier. Homoeopathy has the distinct advantage of being able to "look at the whole patient". So often however, in our ordinary everyday prescribing, this is but a look at the superficial person - the resemblance that fits a remedy - and not an approach that gives an understanding of the whole person, in depth. It has been the aim of this thesis to open up some of these depths.

Appendix A

Effect of homoeopathic treatment in 33 cases studied in depth.

Analysis of effective remedies

Class		Remedies given	
Very good	1.	Thuja 10M Arg. nit 200	Bidor
	2.	Natmur 10M	
	3.	Sulphur 10 M	
	4.	Natmur 200 Aurum per primula	Bidor
	5.	Staphisagria 200, 10M	
	6.	Natmur 200, Ignatia 1M	Bidor
	7.	Kali bich 12	Bidor
	8.	Sulphur 30 Iodum 12	Bidor
	9.	Spigelia 30	
	10.	Sulphur 200 Silicea 200	Bidor
	11.	Arsenicum alb. 10M	Bidor
		Lycopod 10M	
		Bidor 7 Cases	
		Natmur 3 Cases	
		Sulphur 3 Cases	
Good	1.	Natmur 10M	Bidor
	2	Natmur 200, 10M	Bidor
	3.	Phosphorus 30, Sepia 30	
	4.	Medorrhinum IM, Cuprum 30	
	5.	Iris 30 Coffea	
	6.	Sepia 200, Lachesis 30, 200	
	7.	Lycopodium 30, 200 Ignatia 30 Prunus spinoza	
	8.	Sepia 200, Pulsatilla 30	Bidor

Silicea 30

9. Argentum Breap   Bidor
10. Natmur 30, Arsenicum 200   Bidor
11. Phosphorus 200   Bidor
12. Sulphur 10M   Bidor
13. Natmur 30, Thuja 10M
      Bidor (7 cases)
      Natmur (4 cases)
      Sepia (3 cases)

Moderate

1. Spigelia, conium 30
2. Menodorom, Sepia 30 Sulphur 30
3. Medorrhinum Lycopodium 30
    Bromium 10M
4. Arnica 30 Staphisagria 200   Bidor
5. Arnica 30 Silicea 10M Sulphur   Bidor
6. Lycopodium 10M Sulphur 30   Bidor
7. Silicea 30
      Bidor (3 cases)
      Sulphur (3 cases)
      Silicea (2 cases)

No effect

1. Natmur 30, 200 and others
2. Spigelia 6 Pulstilla 10M and others.

Overall reactions of therapy	**Nos.**
Very good	11
Good	13
Moderately good	7
Poor effect	2

These 33 cases were those who answered the invitation to come upto the hospital for an interview concerning their migraine.

124 patients were written to and given an interview appiontment, but only 33 actually managed to come to the hospital. This was a disappointing response.

They do not represent a true cross - section of the out patient material, for those who have benefited from treatment would be more ready to co-operate in a research study than those who have not benefited.

Appendix B provides a study of a truer cross section of all migraine cases that attended Dr. Twentyman's out-patient clinic over a period of 2 years. However, therapeutic effect has only been assessed superficially, from the clinic notes. The disadvantages of such an assessment are fairly obvious.

Appendix B

Assessment of homoeopathic therapy upon 124 cases of migraine based for the most part on a study of the outpatient records.

Overall reactions to threapy	No.
Very good	25
Good	31
Moderately good	20
Poor response	20
(unsuitable for assessment)	28

Of those assessed therefore, 57% showed a good or very good response to homoeopathic therapy.

Analysis of prominent effective remedies

Very good	Bidor	10 cases	(1%)
results	Natmur	5 "	(200m 10M)
	Silicea	3 "	(200)
	Sepia	3 "	(30, 200)
	Lycopodium	3 "	(30, 200)
	Sulphur	3 "	(200, 10M)
Good results	Bidor	13 "	(1%)
	Natmur	9 "	(30, 200, 10M)
	Sepia	5 "	(30, 200)
	Phosphorus	5 "	(30, 200)
	Lachesis	5 "	(30, 200, 10M)

Several remedies are used in the course of treatment of one case and Bidor is almost always used alongside other homoeopathic treatment.

It is, therefore, difficult to dogmatize as to the curative remedy in any one patient though certain remedies recur often amongst the effective group.

Finally, it should be remembered that this analysis pertains to the treatment instituted and carried out mainly by one doctor in one single out-patient department and is not representative of the full therapeutic possibilities available to migraine through Homoeopathy.

Migraine and its Homoeopathic Treatment

Eilhelm Munch MD
Pacific Coast Journal of Homoeopathy
July 1940

1. Arg Nit

Type :   Pronounced neurotic (full of fear and hurry; vertigo and tremors)

Causes : Mental exertion. loss of sleep and body fluids; fright.

Leading symptoms:

(a) Sallow complexion

(b) Craving for sweets, even though they agree poorly; flatulence.

(c) Preferred side or location: left side; especially frontal headache.

(d) Character of headache:

   (i) Boring

   (ii) Pressing

   (iii) Throbbing as if bones of head were pressed asunder

(e) Periodical, come slowly; leave slowly

(f) Abnormal sensation: feeling as if head were enlarged.

Modalities: worse from :-

(a) Warmth (not especially prominent)

(b) Before and during menses

(c) Nights

Better from:-

        (a) pressure, tight bandage

        (b) cold air and cold washing.

Potency: 6X - 30X

2. Belladonna :

        Acts on brain and vessel system (vessel pain)

Type :   Plethoric (strong, full blooded individuals with lively mental faculties, but in severe migraine also sleepy). Especially important in attacks at menstrual times.

Causes:

        (a) overdose of sun

        (b) vexation

        (c) fright

Leading symptoms :

        (a) red, congested face (angio-paralytic migraine)

        (b) preferred side or location: right, over eye, nose, temple

        (c) character of pain: throbbing

        (d) form and kind of attack: periodical, comes and goes suddenly

        (e) abnormal sensations: Wavy pains, as if head should burst, the brain forced out of head and eyes out of their sockets

        (f) eyes sparkle, pupils dilated

        (g) all sense organs are hyper-sensitive; ear; noises; black before eyes.

Modalities:

        (a) Aggravation:

           (i) very sensitive to heat of sun.

(ii) head; colds from hair cutting and drafts

(iii) from motion, especially stooping

(iv) from every touch.

(v) afternoons and evenings

(b) Amelioration:

(i) from cold

(ii) from absolute rest

(iii) sitting upright in darkened room

(iv) covering head

Potency: 6X to 30X

3. Climicifuga racemosa, is closely related to the female organs, their functions or pathalogical, physiological disturbances.

Dysmenorrhoea

Type : Neuropathic, rheumatic

According to Charette: always nervously exhausted, depressed, of pale face with rings around eyes.

According to Donner and Stiegele, for fat women during the climacteric,

Causes : (a) excitement

(b) colds

(c) mental over-exertion

(d) loss of sleep

(e) suppressed menses.

Leading symptoms:

According to Charette: pronounced pale face,

According to Donner: also red cheeked patients.

Side or location: Usually left, above the eye

and temple.

Character of headache:

    (a) boring

    (b) pressing

Character and location of attack

    (a) beginning in neck (arthralgic-myalgic-neuralgic symptoms complex of Donner) extending to front part of head.

    (b) Continued change between physical and psychical complaints.

Abnormal sensations:

changeable, e.g., as if eye were pressed out, or blasting pains at base of skull with sensation of heat on top of head, feeling of cap on head, or as if brain were too large.

Modalities:

    Aggravation: wet, cold weather.

                     Shortly before or at beginning of menses from rest.

    Amelioration:

                     Warm wraps around head, Starting of menses (menstrual headache) From continued easy motion.

Potency : 3X to 6X

4. Coffea, a remedy especially suited to women and children and for the vessel system.

Type: Hypersensitive; hysteria

Causes:

    (a) psychological (joy, fright, unhappy)

    (b) love, quarrel, strife, surprise

    (c) alcohol abuse

(d) chamomilla abuse

Leading symptoms:

 (a) red face

 (b) character of headache : throbbing

 (c) kind of headache; crampy

 (d) abnormal sensation: nail headache

Modalities:

Aggravation: external influences (noise)

     mental emotion

     brain work

     strong scents

     especially nights

Amelioration:

     from lying down, rest

Potency : 3X to 6X

5. Gelsemium.
A great migraine remedy specific in disturbed vision preceding attack.

 Type: Very nervous, irritable (children, women, young people)

 Causes : From emotions, grief, fright (diarrhoea)

 Leading symptoms:

  (a) face dark red

  (b) location: occiput

  (c) character; dull pulsations, disturbed vision before attack (hemianopsy, scotom)

  (d) kind of migraine: periodical, from occiput to vertex or eye

  (e) abnormal sensations: encircling of forehead, head feels "awfully big", stupefaction and confusion.

Modalities:

Aggravation:

(a) motion (nearly all symptoms)

(b) summer heat before change to moist-warm weather

(c) at menstrual time

Amelioration

(a) cool fresh air

(b) stimulants

(c) bending her back

(d) passing much clear urine

Potency: 6X to 30X

6. Glonoine, especially indicated in throbbing vessel pains

Type: Plethoric, sanguine, nervous

Causes :

(a) sun heat

(b) nerve trauma, old scars

(c) hair clipping

(d) suppressed excretions (menses, climacteric)

Leading symptoms:

(a) one-sided redness of face

(b) especially left side

(c) character: strong pulsations, throbbing, hammering

(d) kind: sudden beginning, and leaving with setting sun, from nape of neck upward

(e) abnormal sensations" billowing as from great weight, as if it would press contents

of the skull through forehead, head feels
too big and too full.

Modalities:

Aggravation;

    (a) sun rays

    (b) hot weather

    (c) stopping

    (d) alcohol, especially wine

    (e) quarrel

    (f) mental work

Amelioration;

    (a) from cold, uncovering head

    (b) pressure

    (c) sitting upright

Potency : 6X to 30X

7. Iris versicolor

Type: nervous, gastric. bilious

Causes : from mental overexertion in teachers and
    students.

Leading symptoms:

    (a) pale face

    (b) mostly right-sided, especially eye

    (c) character: intensive throbbing

    (d) Kind: periodical in connection with rest
        periods from hard physical work, especially
        Sunday migraine

    (e) abnormal sensations: Many eye symptoms
        before or at the beginning of the attack
        (migraine ophthalmique of the French
        Blurred vision, hemiopia, blindness, after

burning pain in entire gastro-intestinal
tract (liver and pancreas diseases)

(f) gastric disturbances in the form of violent
acid vomiting at the height of the attack

(g) diarrhoea, light green, bilious

(h) abnormal polyuria follows attack

Modalities:

Aggravation;

(a) hot weather

(b) spring and fall

(c) rest

Amelioration:

(a) from vomiting

(b) from sufficient night sleep

Potency: 6X to 30X

8. Nux vomica is the dyscenesia remedy not only for the
unstriped muscles of the gastrointestinal tract, but also for
the vessels. Angiospastic or angioparalytic migraine with
the vomiting and stomach conditions.

Type : irritable, hypochondriacs of bad temper,
cholerics and neuropathics

Cause:

(a) abuse of alcohol, coffee, spices, tobacco

(b) vexation and worry

(c) mental over-exertion, vigils, business
worries

(d) sexual excesses

(e) sedentary habits

Leading symptoms:

(a) changing complexion (Dark yellow or red,

nervous erethism)

(b) haggard or plethoric stature

(c) location: often left-sided, forehead, occiput

(d) head generally painful

(e) Kind: drilling, pressing, dull

(f) early mornings

(g) abnormal sensations: ineffectual urging to stool; spastic obstipation.

Modalities:

Aggravation;

(a) alcohol, coffee, tobacco

(b) excess in venere

(c) all sensual impressions

(d) mental exertion

(e) cold dry air and winds

Amelioration;

(a) rest

(b) warmth

Potency : 6X to 30X

9. Sanguinaria

Type: pronounced vasomotors (irritable, full of fear)

Causes : Pre-climacteric, menopause

Leading symptoms:

(a) tired expression, head congestion, circumscribed red cheeks

(b) location: above right eyee, forehead

(c) character: throbbing, stitching

(d) Kind: rhythmic, often every 7 days, early morning beginning in nape, extending upwards, locating in region of eyes, rising and falling with sun

(e) abnormal sensations: severe congestions

Modalities:

Aggravation;

(a) noise, light, strong scents

(b) motion

(c) nights in bed

Amelioration:

(a) sleep and darkness

(b) pressure;

(c) vomiting

Potency : 4X

10. Sepia.
Much dependence of the generative phases, especially important in climacteric migraine, i.e, beginning of menopause.

Type :

(a) weakly

(b) fat, irritable, flabby, often apathetic, changing moods, strange changes of character; (egocentric), memory weakness

Cause :

(a) disturbances during climateric

(b) ptoses, especially of uterus and abdominal organs

(c) results of tobacco abuse

Leading symptoms:

(a) sallow complexion, pale, yellow saddle over nose

(b) venous stasis in entire organism (See Puls) especially in portal and female sexual system

(c) desire for sour things

(d) location : left temple, occiput left eye

(e) character: throbbing, stitching, boring

(f) Kind: chronic, spreading forward, from inside out

(g) abnormal sensations:

    (i) frequent congestions with perspiration and vertigo

    (ii) foreign body or ball in different parts of body especially in rectum

    (iii) emptiness in stomach

    (iv) feeling of prolapsus

    (v) thinking of food causes nausea

Modalities:

Aggravation;

    (a) rest in closed rooms

    (b) early morning

    (c) after eating

    (d) during menses

Amelioration;

    (a) exercise, especially in open with exception of those which increase venous states (horse-back riding)

    (b) toward noon and evening

Potency : 6X 30X

11. Spigelia

Type : neuropathic, full of fear

Causes: noises, change of weather, worms.

Leading symptoms:

    (a) pale face from angiospasm.

(b) location: above left eye, especially left
pupil (ciliary neuralgia)

(c) character of pain: sharp, shooting, tearing,
stitching

(d) abnormal sensations : feeling as if head
were open along sagittal suture

Modalities :

Aggravation;

(a) motion

(b) noise

(c) cold air, storm and change of weather

Amelioration;

(a) rest

(b) pressure

(c) head high